asp.

THE NATURAL TREATMENT
OF LIVER TROUBLES

A veteran naturopath explains how liver troubles
are caused and provides detailed advice for
overcoming them naturally and permanently,
without harmful drugs. Principal aim of his
treatment is the elimination of all impurities, a
reaction which can be started by a careful choice
of diet.

The Natural Treatment of Liver Troubles

J. Russell Sneddon N.D.

THORSONS PUBLISHERS LIMITED
Wellingborough, Northamptonshire

First published 1960
Second Impression 1965
Third Impression 1969
Second Edition, revised and reset,
March 1973
Second Impression 1975
Third Impression 1980

ISBN 0 7225 0220 6

Printed and bound in Great Britain by
Hunt Barnard Printing Ltd., Aylesbury, Bucks

Contents

Introduction

MOST OF US have heard the expression: 'He is liverish this morning,' and we take it to mean that such a person is bad-tempered and is best avoided, at least, until he has had his morning coffee. It is very true that a tired and overworked liver can result in its owner becoming melancholic or short-tempered, and it is the purpose of this book to explain how this condition and many other physical and emotional states related to it can be avoided by some health knowledge and a degree of self-control.

It is peculiar, but most of us seem bent on self destruction! We pay so much attention to our clothes and the manner in which we wear them ... to our house and its furnishings ... to our car and our garden. We pry deeply into this and that subject and spend hours studying our hobbies with fervid intensity, but seldom do we study the actions of the body. We eat what we like and never think of the consequences.

Indeed, the people who study their health are regarded as cranks and although occasionally we may be compelled to listen to a dissertation on balanced meals, this is soon dismissed from our minds when appetizing food is on the table. On the subject of food, only one main rule is generally recognized ... eat as much as you can and in any mixture!

It is really amazing that the ordinary man and woman think very little about health — until the appearance of ill-health.

Most people accept their state of health. It may be good ... it may be bad ... but they tend always to accept it without a great deal of questioning. Certainly they may go to the doctor and he is often of great service in diagnosing a certain complaint and in relieving symptoms. The doctor seldom, if ever, goes much deeper than this, and only occasionally does he point out that health, at every stage of life, depends mainly on the actions of the person concerned.

It is very debatable what has been the greatest health discovery of this age, but certainly one of the most important has been the health-giving value of fresh fruit and vegetables. Every doctor is aware of this and there have been several great advertising campaigns to bring this to the public notice. Does the doctor stress this point? No! He would much rather give a bottle of medicine or an injection and leave it to the patient to get well himself. It is not completely correct to blame the doctor because he is forced to do many things which he does not believe in to keep patients on his list. Another point is that explaining about diet takes time and most medical men have little time to spare; anyway, most patients are not interested in diet as a medicine.

This line of reasoning is very wrong because to a great extent we are what we eat and if we wish to attain a certain degree of health then 'good' food must be taken. 'Good' food does not mean food which is cleansed and refined, but food which is as natural as can be obtained and as fresh as possible. Some years ago there was an advertisement which claimed that such and such a product was 'untouched by hand'; with regard to good food it would seem that the motto should be 'untouched by science.' It is now very difficult to obtain natural food which has real health-giving value and this important factor will be stressed throughout this book.

Troubles of the liver and associated organs can be treated and cured by simple methods, but the reader must not conclude that liver trouble is a completely isolated condition. It is not! The whole body is out of rhythm and although the main symptoms may lie in the liver area it is the body as a whole which must be treated. We are whole individuals and cannot entirely single out an organ for special treatment. So what is written in this book may be applied in general to distress in any organ of the body and the reader is advised always to remember that the body must be treated as a whole. The results will often be amazing.

As this book is read it is to be hoped that one point will become apparent — that if we are well it is because we obey nature's laws, and that we become ill, sooner or later, when these laws are violated. Generally, the term violation is used in the physical sense, but the mental aspect is also important. In this respect, fear of the future, of want and ill-health, and fear in general can have a most deleterious effect on health. 'Fear nothing but fear' should be your motto on the way to health.

POSITIVE THOUGHT IS VITAL

Most people who are ill have a poor mental image. They cannot imagine themselves doing great deeds, they feel exhausted at the very thought of physical activity and dread the effect of being forced to carry out certain actions. In this book the methods whereby the physical body can be rejuvenated will be described in detail, and if these are followed they will bring about a great build-up of the physical health. It is essential, however, that this build-up be accompanied by a new conception of the power to do things. A positive bloodstream leads to positive thought, and as the feeling of well-being grows the power to cast out fear becomes stronger. It is excellent to carry always a thought image of what you would like yourself to achieve; a rational and attainable thought-image is the best directive to the physical body. Most people who are suffering pain and discomfort develop a wrong thought image, but as these symptoms are relieved then negative thoughts must be replaced by positive. At first this may appear difficult, but actually it is very easy to think correctly when cleansed and vitalized blood once again courses through the body.

The treatment outlined here is based on the belief that there is within the body an inherent healing power. The methods employed are calculated to enable this healing power to operate to its fullest extent and thus enable the person to be restored to full strength.

This is real Nature Cure treatment, drugless, in that no form of medication is used, but whatever the methods employed the basic principle is that it is the internal healing power which really does the work. Thus the water applications, the exercises, the diet and all other methods advised are prescribed for the purpose of strengthening this internal power which is, to a greater or lesser degree, within each of us.

The question then arises that if this healing power is resident within the body how is it that we become ill? That is a fair question. Actually from early childhood the healing power of the body has been showing its presence. It shows itself first of all by acute disturbances of the health in the form of fevers, sickness, catarrhal discharges, lack of appetite – in fact, by a whole host of symptoms which generally mean that the little body has become congested and ill at ease. The healing power develops the sickness and uses the loss of appetite and consequent symptoms to rid itself of its encumbrances. So far so good, and if the child is fasted, rested and perhaps given compresses if the fever is very high, then the result will be a freshened and invigorated body. That is the Nature Cure way of treating acute disease and it is a very sensible and successful way which ensures that the child never becomes really congested and chronically ill.

Unfortunately very few children are treated by such methods and even in the very simple children's ailments some form of medication is given – perhaps the common aspirin or some more complicated drug. The result is that the healing power of the body is thwarted. If this is continued the ill-health of childhood deepens into the ill-health of early adult life when the troubles are much more deep-rooted. Even then, however, the throwing-off tendency of the person with inherent vital strength is not recognized; and such is the prevailing system of medicine in this country that drugs must be given whenever some physical upset arises. Thus, in one way, the natural healing power of the body is weakened and does not exert its full force.

Another way is that the food that the child and young adult usually receive is not natural and balanced, and substances are introduced into the bloodstream which can prove harmful if not quickly eliminated. In other words, most of the population of this country are not fed on the lines which ensure a perfectly healthy body, with normal recuperative power.

At this point it can be argued that the healing power is not dependent upon food, but it is common sense that it is much more likely that healing power or vitality is more potent in healthy than in diseased tissues.

So the suppression of acute cleansing actions and poor food have their effect in producing ill-health which cannot always be controlled by inherent healing power. There are other factors, such as poor hereditary tendencies, environmental and occupational conditions, all of which require study, although in these respects the general up-lifting of our standard of living has done excellent work in the past decade or two. From the naturopathic standpoint it is a great pity that the basic factor of health, namely, the supply of balanced and non-toxic food, has not made similar progress.

In this book will be outlined a system of health understanding based on the proved working of the human body. There is some healing vitality in even the very weak person and if it can be vitalized by thought, food and knowledge, then some degree of cure can nearly always be obtained.

At the same time it is not the purpose of this book to make the reader a faddist on health matters. Common sense and co-operation with the body's desires are the basis of real health and the unattainable is not promised. Yet if there is a measure of healing vitality present it can be so released that miracles of healing may often be obtained. These have occurred many times, surprising both patient and practitioner alike.

A health magazine at one time carried the axiom, 'The Release of Health for the Joy of Living,' and that phrase sums up our case very thoroughly. In most patients health is waiting to be released. It is our stubbornness, our lack of health knowledge which makes a comparatively easy action seem so difficult. Everyone is anxious to be well. The body is anxious to work efficiently. All that is needed is to remove the brakes.

To do this, however, it is necessary to replace old habits by new ones, and in doing so we must deny ourselves certain things which appear to be indispensable. Actually they only appear so because once they are done without their importance is seen in its true light.

Once started on the real road to health it will soon be appreciated that many things happen to supplement our ideas. Within a few weeks it is common to find that a completely new feeling prevails throughout the body. The carriage is more erect and there is a general feeling of confident radiation which is always lacking in the ill person. This is quickly realized by friends, who remark about the change although unaware of the methods being used to regain health.

Health does not come back suddenly. It spreads from cell to cell and the speed of cure depends on cell vitality. To this end the main aim of treatment is the elimination of all impurities, a reaction which can be started by a careful choice of diet.

I.
Talking about Food

IT IS PRESUMED that you are reading this book because your health is not ideal and it is likely that the trouble is associated with liver or some kindred ailment. From the Nature Cure standpoint there is, as has been stated before, only *one* disease — that is, general ill-health of varying degrees of intensity. Therefore we must break into the cycle which has been explained in the previous chapter to prevent the further decline of health. The best way to do this is by diet, and your body starts rejuvenating immediately it is given *real* food. By this is meant food which supplies the body with everything it requires and leaves very little surplus. Before going more deeply into the subject matter of this book it would be most helpful if in this chapter we studied some of the basic principles of Nature Cure to enable the reader to begin healing right away by a few simple dietetic adjustments of a general nature.

The very first point that should be stressed is that you locate the nearest health food store and become a customer. These stores keep the best foods, as much as possible unadulterated and usually the vegetables and fruits supplied are compost-grown. This means that the ground on which the food is grown is fed by natural means, such as the compost heap, with the addition of lime and other minerals which are known to be natural to the soil. Nature Cure practitioners believe that food formed in growth by artificial fertilizers is unbalanced food. It follows that when this is eaten it introduces substances foreign to the human body, causing peculiar upsets. There are many health food stores in this country and they should be supported in their efforts to bring wholesome food within our reach. The vitamin-mineral salt content of food is of great importance and the person who has a garden can do much for his health by growing food naturally. There are many books, packed with vital information, on this subject.

In this way it is possible to ensure that at least some of the food taken is pure and this is a most important step towards health. Freshly gathered vegetables have a different taste altogether and, what is more important, they are better than bought vegetables because the vitamin content has not had time to deteriorate. It is from the vegetable world that we also gain some very important mineral salts, and in a person in poor health it is probable that these minerals will be deficient or at least that the body will be incapable of utilizing them. The home gardener, by following the compost method of feeding the soil and by choosing the vegetables which can be eaten raw does much to improve the quality and 'life' of this food. Vitamins necessary for the chemical reactions within the body are then easily obtained and the quality is much better. It is the quality of food which is lacking today.

It has been said that many people have plenty of minerals in their body but cannot use them. This is correct in certain cases, but the large majority of people have a definite need for certain mineral salts. This is shown in lifeless hair, blotched and scaly skin and poor teeth, which never seem to harden and which are removed surgically at an early age. Impaired sight and a poor condition of the surroundings of the eyes is often the result of deficiency. Stomach and bowels require minerals to maintain their tone and to remove the very common digestive upsets. Many, many instances can be quoted regarding the signs of mineral deficiency.

It is possible, of course, to supply the body with plenty of good minerals and yet find that assimilation of them is very slow. This is only a part of the re-education of the body. It must first of all be clean in the assimilative parts and the specialized cells of the small bowel must be retained to abstract the needed minerals from the food. When this function is normalized — and it may take months to achieve it — one of the first changes to be noticed will be in the nails. These will become thicker, stronger, less ridged and less liable to breakage. All longitudinal and transverse markings will disappear. The advancement of new health can be judged to a large extent by the nails and all readers following Nature Cure methods are advised to study their own nails and note the beneficial reaction.

RAW VEGETABLES FOR HEALTH

Next in importance to the need for ensuring that our food is well grown, is its preparation. To obtain and maintain health a supply of raw vegetables and fruit each day is the ideal way of getting vitamins and minerals. Naturally there are objections to this because some people cannot under any circumstance, digest raw food, although it is possible that this ability may be developed as real health returns. Other people who have deficient teeth cannot chew uncooked food. This difficulty can be minimized by grating vegetables and fruits very finely or by using one of the mechanical pulverizers to obtain the pulp of the vegetable and its juice. In passing it must be stressed that poor, deficient teeth must be treated. The introduction in one way or another of raw vegetables and fruit daily does much to maintain the chemical balance of the blood. Such a meal can be made very appetizing when tastefully arranged. It will not increase the weight, but it does increase the health.

Over-cooking of vegetables is the most common fault and such vegetables, in addition to being distasteful, are practically useless as food. Here are the important points which must be observed:

First of all, cast-steel or heavy enamel pans should be used for cooking and the use of aluminium utensils should be avoided.

Steam the vegetables, using as little water as possible. Vitamins and minerals are always lost during cooking, but the loss is minimized by this method. The vegetable water should be used in the preparation of soup. Coarse vegetables should be chopped or shredded before cooking and potatoes should be baked in their skins.

Nature Cure has been called 'the salad-a-day diet' and we believe that everyone would be healthier if they could obtain a raw salad every day of the year. Most people think of salad as lettuce and tomato, but nowadays it is possible to get some form of salad right through the winter.

Salads contain vitamins and a plentiful supply of mineral salts, although they actually have little 'fuel' value. In other words, their purpose is to supply salts which are necessary for perfect health, at least, in most people. There are, of course, many instances of people who live into the eighties in good health and who have never had a salad or, indeed, who have had very little cooked vegetables. These people are blessed with a goodly supply of residual mineral salts from which they can draw at will and which does not seem to need any great replenishing. Most of us, however, have not got this supply; we have to introduce salts every day if we wish to maintain health and the salad is the best source of these salts.

As the salad is uncooked, we need an efficient system of mastication, so the teeth should be checked carefully. Many people lose one tooth at a time and often the grinders are completely missing. These people then attempt to chew their food with their front teeth and this is seldom, if ever, satisfactory and ill-health can often be traced to inadequate mastication.

Thorough chewing of food is most important. It aids stomach and intestinal digestion and prepares the stomach for the food. It stimulates bowel action and this is further aided by the bulk of the salad meal. This bulk provides the best of all roughage and forms a plug of cellulose fibres which cleans the *villi* of the intestinal canal and helps assimilation.

Although most people think of salad based on lettuce and tomatoes, these are not the really important foods. Lettuce must be grown quickly to be crisp (cos lettuce is always the best) and it has not time to extract a full quota of salts from the soil. Long-growing vegetables, such as brussels sprouts, cabbage, greens and main-crop potatoes, are very rich in these salts and are much more beneficial than the quick-growing salads. All vegetables, however, should be used freely and they can be mixed with fruit or fruit juice to make the salad more interesting.

Once you have made up your mind to improve your health by taking a salad each day do not spoil it by introducing a salad dressing based on vinegar. Take lemon juice only and if this proves upsetting to the stomach, mix it with a little olive oil.

At this stage the reader may wonder when he is going to start curing trouble of the liver or any other organ in this vicinity. If he has obeyed the advice given in this chapter he has already started his cure. Make no mistake about 'cures.' You cannot make another person well by giving him this or that. You can stimulate his healthy vitality and this makes him well by harnessing many healing methods. Basically, however, we are to a very great extent dependent on the type of food we eat and if the above advice is followed, then the body will begin to assimilate the foods that are required for health.

2.
What the Liver Does

NOW THAT CERTAIN important food rules have been laid down, and, it is to be hoped, studied and followed by the reader so that healing can be commenced, we can go deeper into the subject of liver troubles. It is necessary at this point to give a rough idea of the functions of the digestive system to enable the reader to follow the principles outlined in this book. The accompanying diagram (see next page) explains how this system is arranged.

Food after mastication in the mouth passes to the stomach, which is actually a large storage bag. In it the food is subjected to the action of the juices excreted from the stomach walls. This digestion continues for a certain time, depending on the type of food, and then the contents of the stomach are acted upon by a fluid called bile, which passes upwards from the duodenum. Shortly afterwards the contents of the stomach are passed downwards into the duodenum, which is actually the first part of the small bowel. All this interchange takes place automatically and is outside our control.

In the duodenum, digestion of the food is continued and the bowel itself gives a juice to aid this process. By stimulation, the bile from the liver and the pancreatic juice from the pancreas also flow into the duodenum to aid the digestion. The bile comes from the liver and is passed down the common bile duct. It is stored in the gall-bladder when not required. When, however, the food is about to enter the duodenum from the stomach, the gall-bladder forces the bile downwards into the small bowel and it is the flowing bile which stimulates the pancreatic action.

The liver is one of the most important organs of the body. It is mainly situated on the right side under the lower ribs and its edge can often be felt if the fingers are inserted beneath the ribs at the front of the body and pressure is made in an upward direction. In certain liver ailments the organ swells and then it comes well down below the rib margin, but in still other liver conditions the organ shrinks and becomes small and very hard. There is a saying in medical circles that 'when the liver is small then

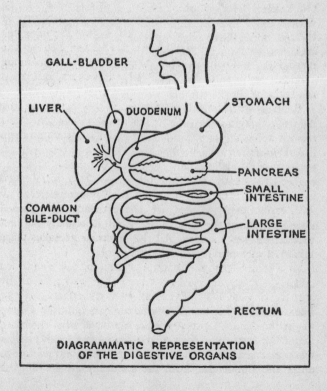

DIAGRAMMATIC REPRESENTATION
OF THE DIGESTIVE ORGANS

you feel well,' but actually the liver can be too small for perfect health. It is a large, heavy organ weighing about three-and-a-half pounds and usually contains about a quarter of the blood in the body. In this respect it really acts as a reservoir from which blood can be drawn and sent to any part of the body which requires it. This reaction is very speedy indeed and again is automatic.

The liver consists of many millions of tiny cells, vessels and small ducts. Its main purpose is to deal with blood, which contains a complicated mixture of food, impurities and toxins. The purpose of the liver cells is to pick and choose, retaining the food and expressing the impurities and toxins. Between the cells, in addition to the blood vessels, are formed small collecting tubes which gradually enlarge until they make up the large tube called the common bile duct. This bile duct is connected to the duodenum, but along its length is the gall-bladder, which acts as a storehouse for bile, when it is not required for digestion or for the stimulation of the bowel. Bile also acts as a laxative. The flow of bile, as has been mentioned before, stimulates the flow of juice from the pancreas and this also aids digestion, especially that of fatty food. The liver also stores sugar in the form of glycogen, and when extreme muscular activity takes place this glycogen is changed back into sugar and sent to the muscles requiring it.

The duodenum is the first part of the small intestine where most of the nutrients from digested food are transferred into the bloodstream. The vessels which gather this food then pass it to the liver.

ACTION OF THE LIVER

The action of the liver is very complicated and in a book of this kind only a rough outline can be given of the more important actions which take place when the liver is working. Most of the food and other substances which are introduced into the digestive tract during the normal course of living are sent through the wall of the small intestine and eventually reach the liver.

After this many reactions are performed. Protein foods such as meat, eggs, cheese, beans, lentils, nuts, etc., are broken up and used to renew tissues and to provide energy. The end products of protein digestion are prepared by the liver into certain more simple substances, which are eliminated by the kidneys. Starchy and sugary foods, on the other hand, are broken down in the liver and changed into glycogen, which is retained in the liver but is available immediately to any part of the muscular system which requires this energy-giving sugar.

Impurities, which are present in every type of food, are isolated by the liver and eliminated through the organs designed for this purpose, but first of all they are changed into harmless substances by being detoxicated. An active liver is therefore the best safeguard against all forms of food poisoning and, indeed, any kind of poisoning.

In the liver, old blood cells are broken down and the iron content which is essential to their efficiency is taken out and arranged in such a way that it can again be used in new blood cells. The cell envelope is taken away and used in the formation of the bile. This bile is then sent down the common bile duct and stored in the gall-bladder until such times as it is needed for digestion or for the stimulation of the bowel, because the bile is actually the natural laxative of the body. It will be easily understood that, if for any reason the bile becomes too concentrated, the flow becomes sluggish and the formation of bile-stones is imminent.

As has been said before, the flow of bile stimulates the action of the pancreas, and the liver and pancreas work together in health. This is one of the reasons why the Nature Cure practitioner believes that in certain pancreatic diseases, such as diabetes, the action of the liver is very important.

Bile is also most useful in controlling the acidity of the stomach, and liver troubles are common causes of gastric and duodenal ulcerations, as explained in a companion book on that subject.

SERIOUS LIVER CHANGES

Troubles of the liver are complex and various because of the numerous functions performed by this organ. For instance, the liver receives two blood supplies, namely, venous blood from the portal vein and arterial blood from the hepatic artery. This is one of the weaknesses of the liver, because any disturbance of the circulation, such as thrombosis, of either of these two supplies can result in very serious liver changes. In this modern age the clotting of the blood circulation is all too common and the liver often suffers in this way. This is explained in greater detail later in this book.

The liver is greatly dependent on good nutritional facilities, and a poor protein diet with a high fat content is dangerous to the liver function if indulged in over a prolonged period. A relatively high protein diet is essential to liver health.

Most of us think that alcohol and liver troubles are associated and it is interesting to find that investigation does not bear out this contention. It is admitted that cirrhosis of the liver is more common to alcoholics than abstainers. There are, of course, nutritional factors which come into this and the person who drinks heavily is often a very heavy eater.

LIVER TROUBLES IN PREGNANCY

On the subject of nutrition, a factor which seldom receives much attention is the frequency with which pregnant women suffer from liver troubles. Undoubtedly the demands of the growing foetus are often only satisfied at the expense of the mother's strength and there must be adequate compensation in the diet. It is certain that many people who follow the Nature Cure tenets are not fully conversant with this need and the amount of protein taken during pregnancy is often too small, because the woman may not have a high assimilative rhythm. This is often shown by the fact that the woman does not lay down more fat than normal during her pregnancy.

The liver can be adversely affected by chemicals and also by the excessive use of tea, mushrooms, etc., and is definitely harmed by phosphorus and chloroform. Physiologically it is important to note that oxygen in the blood is also needed in quantity to ensure health in the liver.

The most helpful way of giving advice on liver troubles is to take the more common conditions separately and describe in some detail how they can be corrected by simple, natural methods. This, of course, is not the ideal, because in Nature Cure we believe that there is only one real disease, although it has many forms of manifestation, and that a basic treatment covers all conditions.

3.
Simple Liver Enlargement

ONE OF THE most common ailments of the liver is termed simple liver enlargement. It occurs in varying degrees of intensity and has the following symptoms:

There is a peculiar sense of fulness on the right side of the body, around the lower ribs, usually accompanied by pain and a feeling of oppression when the area is pressed. Many sufferers feel well when they are resting, but on rising and attaining the upright position, feel rather sick, with a great sense of weight in the liver area.

Usually there are changes in the complexion, which is often very pale and even assumes a rather dusky hue. The tongue is coated, furred and generally yellow in colour, although in severe cases it may appear to be greenish. The bowel is constipated and the person feels that if an adequate bowel movement could be obtained then all would be well. Headache is another common feature in simple liver congestion and it may be accompanied by vomiting, which generally relieves the condition. The pulse is slow and often irregular.

Causes – In many cases the trouble is brought on by a sudden chill and undoubtedly if the feet become very cold then it is possible for the blood temperature of the lower limbs to fall and the liver can become chilled very easily. It is unlikely, however, that a very healthy liver would be affected in this way and usually there has been some previous difficulty.

The general and most common cause is a too-high protein and fat diet, including eggs, meat, fried fish, excessive butter and margarine and other fried and greasy foods. Alcohol and wines also engorge the liver, although not so much as is commonly imagined. Excessive consumption of sweets containing unbalanced and synthetic sweetening agents is also very upsetting to this organ.

In most cases people overeat of the protein, fatty and sugary foods, but they do it for so long that it becomes a habit and undoubtedly the liver can, within reason, adapt itself to very trying conditions. In other cases, however, the person is aware that his liver is very sensitive and will not stand overloading, and such people tend to watch their diet. When the blood does become overloaded the usual 'cure' is to take a liver pill and within a few days everything seems as good as ever. Putting too much strain on the liver, however, whether occasional or habitual, does harm the organ and as the years pass it becomes increasingly difficult for the person to feel really well. He may have short spells in which his health appears to be good, but most days he has periods in which he cannot tell what is wrong, but feels sluggish, depressed and his digestive system is uneasy. A peculiar form of constipation often affects these people. One day their bowel is working well. Next day there is complete cessation of movement and then comes diarrhoea. This is due to an interruption in the flow of bile, which is the natural laxative for the bowel and it often occurs when the liver becomes congested.

Treatment — It does not matter how severe the attack is, the treatment should be on the following lines: First of all a complete fast is indicated, taking nothing but water. Warm water is usually best because it seems to stimulate the flow of bile. At the same time, if the patient desires cold water, then this is allowed. If the water invokes sickness this is quite helpful and will relieve the condition quickly. If the trouble is extensive and the feeling of liver congestion is severe then the alternate hot and cold packs, advised later in this book, should be used over the liver area. These stimulate the drainage of the part and help greatly in reducing the swollen organ.

It is not likely that the tongue will clear within two days and so the fast should be extended as long as possible. Frequently this results in a more widespread headache, but the patient should not resort to aspirin, but should take nothing but water. During this time the bowel may not work, but nothing should be done unless there is actual bowel pain, when a warm-water enema may be taken to relieve the flatulence, which is the usual cause.

Once the acute symptoms have abated then a meal or two of fruit only should be taken. Sweet apples, pears, grapes and fruit juice are the most suitable and they may be taken in any quantity. The fruit is cleansing and antiseptic and will aid bowel action. The fruit diet should be continued until there is a feeling that a more solid meal can be taken. This period varies with the intensity of the attack and it may be several days before the liver and bowel are sufficiently relieved to take more food. When it does occur the diet should be built on the following lines:

Breakfast — Any type of wheat-germ with a small amount of unpasteurized milk. If more roughage is required for bowel action, then all-bran cereal may be added. Soaked prunes, figs or raisins. One or two slices of rough wholewheat toast. Butter or vegetarian margarine should be used sparingly. To drink — cereal coffee, yeast extract.

If, however, it is found that the fruit breakfast alone is sufficient then this may be taken in place of the above, with or without a glass of whole milk. Between meals water is allowed if there is actual thirst and this usually occurs if there is any tendency to liver congestion.

Lunch — If this is the main protein meal then a small amount of lean meat or steamed or baked fish or cheese pudding or a lightly-cooked egg may be taken. The meat should be limited to once weekly, fish once weekly and only two eggs per week. Vegetarian savouries may be taken to replace the meat and fish course if desired. With the protein take two steamed root vegetables and baked, jacketed potatoes.

Dessert — The best dessert is fruit of any kind (except tinned fruit), but occasionally a brown rice pudding or milk junket may be taken. Many people feel the need for vegetable soup during the winter months. There is really nothing against this, but it should contain a large amount of vegetable and not too much water. This meal should be taken as dry as possible to allow mastication to be complete.

The Third Meal — The sufferer from frequent attacks of liver congestion should take a very simple third meal. A salad is the best basis. Use as many green and grated root vegetables as obtainable and also sweet fruits, such as apples, pears and dates. No salad dressing, except a little lemon juice, because olive oil is often too heavy for liverish people. Follow with wholewheat bread or crisp-bread, with a small amount of unsalted butter or vegetarian margarine and a little honey.

Supper — If supper is desired, then it should be limited to fruit or fruit juice.

In this trouble great attention must be paid to the control of protein foods, namely, meat, fish, eggs, peas, beans, lentils, nuts and milk. These foods definitely throw strain on the liver and any person subject to repeated attacks of liver congestion must limit the proteins in the diet to one per day. Even then, if meat is taken, all fat must be removed. Fish must be steamed or baked, never fried. Eggs can be taken raw with orange juice or lightly boiled or poached and limited to two per week. All fats must also be taken in small amounts and limited to unsalted butter, vegetarian margarine — a very small helping of nut or olive oil.

It is not always possible in our social life to avoid heavy meals or, indeed, a succession of such meals and the person who suffers from liver congestion must select his food very carefully on these occasions. If it is felt that the liver has been overworked, a day's fast or a fruit day will generally rest the liver and renew its function. Resting the liver is preferable to the artificial stimulation of the liver pill, although in many cases it is actually the more difficult 'medicine' to take.

When the liver action inclines to be sluggish it is also a very good plan to have a fruit day, taking no other food, once per month. This also prevents many people from suffering liver congestion.

IMPORTANCE OF EXERCISE

Modern life leads to many illnesses of inactivity and without doubt the liver suffers often in this connection. Active exercise provides an adequate supply of oxygen in the blood and makes the work of the liver so much easier. It also stimulates the blood and venous flow and many forms of sport and physical movement bring about a self-massage of the liver itself. In the chapter on exercise in this book, certain exercises beneficial to liver health are described and they should be practised carefully each day.

People who are not naturally indolent feel the need for exercise, otherwise their bodies become sluggish and they do not feel well. These are signs of lack of oxygen and engorgement of the liver, and careful dieting and exercise is the remedy. The old-fashioned but very helpful walk in the evening is now replaced by a car run or bus tour and the digestive organs suffer every time. This is why people say they are in better health when they are working. It is the exercise which stimulates the liver action.

So whenever possible obtain a short walk in the morning and evening and treat it as a health-giving exercise. It need not be long, from five to ten minutes being sufficient to bring about the movement of blood required to prevent engorgement.

4.
Bowel Catarrh or Mucous Colitis

NATURE CURE METHODS, on which this book is based, are always directed at treating the body as a whole in the belief that it is impossible for one organ by itself to go completely wrong. It is admitted that symptoms often point to the inefficiency of one part, but closer investigation will prove that other and frequently nearby organs are also affected. At the same time we must begin treatment somewhere and usually this is directed at relieving the organ which is not working correctly. To a certain extent, this is giving in to the desires of the patient, but it is not always a bad thing, nor one which can be avoided.

The first condition to be studied is that of bowel catarrh or more medically, mucous colitis. This is an ailment which ultimately affects the liver or which can result from the overloading of that organ, so it becomes an important study.

Catarrh in any form is a sign that the body is choked. It is the most common of all conditions, although it is often not recognized as such because disease is indivisible. Catarrh means that one or more of the following conditions has arisen:

1. Food has been taken in excess of the body's requirements.
2. The food has been of very poor quality.
3. There is a lack of certain mineral salts.

4. It is likely that the eliminating organs have become overworked.

Let us study these points in some detail because they offer great guidance in health matters.

Too much food means that the person either suffers from a very healthy appetite and has made no attempt to curb it or else the body has created a false hunger. The person with the very healthy appetite must burn up the food with physical activity or else flesh is laid down.

This increase in weight is abnormal and it means that the tissues are in some distress due to the storing of the unwanted food. Ultimately this excessive food mass forms the actual catarrh. Food which is not used for its proper purpose always becomes dangerous to the body and for this reason under-eating is always to be preferred to over-eating if there is any sign of catarrh.

POOR FOOD CREATES CATARRH

The second point, that of the person suffering from catarrh due to eating food of poor quality, is also very common. The outstanding examples of this kind of food are all white-flour products, white sugar and pasteurized milk. These foods (and here milk is regarded as a solid food) are unbalanced and upset the chemistry of the blood. White flour products are particularly harmful because, with the addition of fluid, they form a paste which clogs the tissues, especially of the bowel, giving rise to the familiar catarrhal discharge.

All food introduced into the body should satisfy the requirement that it builds and repairs tissues or gives heat and energy and does not require much elimination. The foods mentioned above do not do this because they are not in their true state and have been rendered unnatural by processing. In addition to the common classification of food such as protein, carbohydrates and fats, Nature Cure thought has continually stressed that to balance and neutralize these foods, a continual supply of mineral-salt-containing foods is necessary. The best source of these salts is the vegetable kingdom and raw vegetables each day become a necessity in this modern world. When the salts are missing, then certain important chemical reactions do not take place. For instance, the full utilization of starchy food is such a reaction and if one particular salt is missing, this means that catarrhal material is easily formed and ultimately the person displays all the symptoms of this trouble.

The fourth point emphasizes that the eliminating organs of the body, namely, the skin, kidneys, lungs and bowel, are not equal to the task of dealing with the unwanted material, otherwise catarrh would not arise. To be healthy a balance must be set up with regard to the amount of unwanted material retained within the system.

Catarrh then is a collection of unwanted substances within the tissues of the body. It is natural that the intelligence of the cells becomes disturbed at its presence and sends it to the organs of elimination, and some of it is expelled. Usually, however, these organs are not fit to deal with extra amounts and the remainder is stored in some safe place such as the sinuses of the face, the scalp, in the outer layers of the skin, in the bronchial tubes, and so on.

Notice that these organs are all surface tissues and that the catarrhal material can be easily removed when conditions are perfect. So far so good, and if the gradual throw-out of material is allowed to continue, a healthy balance is struck. If the person realizes what is happening, and this means understanding the underlying principles of Nature Cure, the body can be helped in its endeavours by fasting and other measures, and then real health will result. This unfortunately is not always the case, and then the following sequence of suppression is common.

EFFECTS OF SUPPRESSION

Pain in the facial sinuses, a catarrhal condition, is generally treated by drugs to kill the pain, by surgical draining to wash out the part if it is accessible and by strong applications of heat. The catarrh is thus driven to some deeper tissue.

Catarrh of the scalp in its elimination causes the condition known as dandruff and because by this time the catarrhal material is becoming acidic, it results in lifeless hair with a tendency to baldness. Naturally the sufferer does not appreciate what is happening and he vigorously applies one of the many preparations which are reputed to 'cure' dandruff. Many of these so-called cures are of a poisonous nature and once again the catarrh is suppressed and the effort of the body to throw it out through the scalp ducts is thwarted.

Catarrh of the bronchial tubes causes the condition known as bronchitis and a very serious one it can become, but if it is treated in the primary stage as a symptom or a sign that the body is trying to eliminate foreign impurity then it can be easily cured. Unfortunately this is seldom the case and most physicians look upon bronchitis as a symptom which must be removed immediately, with the result that again the out-throw of impurity is thrust further into the tissues of the body. We could go on explaining how the signs of catarrh on the surface of the body are generally treated by measures which ultimately result in the catarrh going deeper into the tissues and joints and into the vital parts of the organism.

SYMPTOMS OF BOWEL CATARRH

We have, however, said enough to enable the reader to understand that catarrh of the bowel is seldom a primary condition. It is generally the result of some suppression of a catarrhal outlet and is therefore of a secondary nature. It is also a more serious condition than one which shows its signs on the surface of the body. Bowel catarrh, or mucous colitis, as it is called, is common between the ages of twenty and forty, and is much more frequently found in females. Generally there is a definite loss of weight and the person becomes thin, has a poor appetite, there is anaemia and very often, if the normal fat is lost, some prolapse of the abdominal organs. All this results in the woman's life becoming very uncertain and in most cases nervous symptoms appear, and we have a very temperamental woman inclined often to be melancholic with a very poorly nourished body.

There are periods in which the bowel seems to work fairly normally. These are called the 'periods of freedom' and this condition may last for months, even up to six months, although the health during this time is never perfect. The attacks themselves vary from a few days to several months, and it is usually possible to trace the onset of an attack to some definite error in diet, although it often reacts after some high emotional tension. The common symptoms are first of all a very obstinate constipation, but peculiarly enough there may be sudden attacks of diarrhoea. Often the patient suffers from a form of colic with considerable stress in the bowel, and a great deal of mucus is passed with the bowel motion. Casts of the bowel are often found in the stools and bleeding is another symptom.

The condition is a very depressing one, but it is rarely fatal and responds to treatment. Although there is a tendency to recurrence, many cases are cured permanently. A full range of Nature Cure treatment is required in chronic cases. The bowel must be strengthened and any prolapse corrected by manipulation and systematic exercise. In severe cases an abdominal belt may be required. A weight gain is a good sign, but it must be obtained from healthful, balanced food. Sufferers become alarmed when an attack commences and they tend to eat too many of the bland foods such as starches and milk in an effort to stop the inflammation within the irritated bowel. As has been stated, this condition is of a catarrhal nature and to add more catarrhal material in an effort to soothe is not ultimately beneficial.

In chronic colitis the condition is always difficult

because the liver and gall-bladder actions are usually very temperamental. The basis of the treatment should be to take non-roughage food when the condition is active and the following type of diet is indicated:

Breakfast — Slippery elm food and milk.

Lunch — Starchy food with bananas and milk.

Evening Meal — Egg or cheese dish with starch and milk.

In severe cases the milk diet itself is often necessary. In this diet milk is taken in small quantities every hour or two and during the whole day quite a considerable amount may be taken. This diet should be continued when the colitis is active, but although it is soothing it is not healing. Stop it as soon as possible, replacing it with a more balanced diet such as:

Breakfast — Prunes or stewed apples or pears.

Lunch — Egg or cheese dish with one steamed vegetable. Whole-rice pudding.

Evening Meal — Wholewheat starch with tomatoes or fruit.

Gradually, as the condition improves, put in more and more vegetables and fruit, but always avoid flesh protein and fish.

Usually a tolerance for the roughage diet will be gained, but for many months trial and error in diet must be practised and no set rules can be given because each case is different.

5.
Jaundice

JAUNDICE IS ONE of the most common conditions associated with the liver and when it occurs many sufferers become gravely concerned, believing it means that a more serious disease is present. In most cases, however, the trouble is of a comparatively simple origin and recourse to Nature Cure treatment should bring about a rapid and progressively heartening change.

The most common exciting cause of jaundice is eating an unbalanced and too heavy meal. This is readily understood when a number of general diets are studied and most Nature Cure practitioners wonder why it is that the patient has been able to withstand, without upset, these excesses for so many years. The basic causes of jaundice can be gall-stones which are blocking the common bile duct; the presence of foreign bodies in this canal; or a thickening of the bile. Another common condition associated with mucous colitis (described in the previous chapter), is that of catarrhal inflammation of the common bile duct.

There is also a more severe form of jaundice termed 'toxic jaundice,' but in this condition there is high fever with delirium and occasionally convulsions. In this serious form, suppression of urine is common and small red haemorrhages may arise all over the skin.

Jaundice need not be completely associated with the physical state of the body, but may be induced by severe mental shock, prolonged emotional strain or even by a sudden bout of anger. In these emotional conditions it is believed that the bile ducts are thrown into spasm and create a back pressure towards the liver and gall-bladder.

The most common form of jaundice is catarrhal jaundice. Usually here some form of catarrh is already present and an exciting cause such as a heavy meal is only required to upset the condition. Now, as has been stated before, catarrh in the system shows that food supplied is not fully utilized by the body and the residues become catarrhal deposits. Stomach catarrh, due mainly to food indiscretion, is most common and many peculiar feelings can be due to its presence. Generally this condition at one time or another affects the duodenum, and, as will be seen from the diagram, the common bile duct enters the duodenum and catarrhal inflammation can spread from the small bowel into the bile duct. This is the most common of all causes of jaundice and in most cases the catarrh is already present and some dietetic indiscretion sets up the inflammation.

THE SYMPTOMS OF CATARRHAL JAUNDICE

A brownish discoloration of the skin appears which usually, but not always becomes itchy. Closer examination will show that the whites of the eyes have a yellowish tinge and there is also some darkening in the colour of the soft palate. It is common to find that the bowel motion becomes clay coloured and in most cases there is also a change in the colour of the urine. On physical examination the liver is usually found to be enlarged and tender on palpation, the pulse is frequently slow, often abnormally so, and the patient is languid, sleepy and very disinclined for mental effort. In other cases, the patient becomes definitely melancholic or extremely irritable. In passing, it may be stated that these symptoms in varying degree are all common signs of liver trouble. In simple catarrh of the liver there is usually little pain and no emaciation. The discoloration of the skin lasts according to the severity of the attack; frequently it will be gone completely within a week, but in other cases it may last for several weeks.

TREATMENT

During the acute attack the patient should be fasted and if possible this should be continued until the heavily coated and rather foul tongue becomes clean. Such a fast again depends upon the underlying cleanliness of the system and when a bloodstream has become very dirty such a long fast would be called for that it may be impossible to continue it until the tongue becomes clean. If, however, the patient feels that he must break his fast, then fresh fruit and fruit juices should be taken. With regard to the type of fruit, it is difficult to lay down hard and fast rules. Actually the desires of the patient are a good guide, but in most cases it will be found that bananas, being a starchy type of food, are not suitable and oranges may not agree, although there have been cases in which the desire for oranges has been intense. Fruit juice and warm water should be the only drinks and the patient should continue for as long as he can on this fruit and juice diet, because each day means that the liver is rested, that the bowel catarrh is reduced and the body is given the ideal opportunity of retoning and cleansing its tissues.

When the desire for more solid food becomes over-riding, then steamed and raw vegetables with starch in the form of a baked potato should be given and the patient should continue along these lines until another change of food becomes necessary. Then wholewheat starches may be introduced and it will be seen that the protein foods — meat, fish, peas, beans, lentils, cheese and milk, are the last foods along with fats to be reintroduced.

These are the foods which throw great strain on the liver and therefore they must be taken in strict moderation if the organ has to be rested. There are many authorities who believe — and there is considerable evidence on this score — that meat dishes do stimulate certain glands of the liver. I can only say that the person who suffers from jaundice of a recurring nature would be advised to study whether his diet should contain a little meat or should be completely vegetarian. There are points on both sides, but it appears that much more harm is done through the over-eating of meat than through its too-limited use.

In severe cases of jaundice the liver area – that is the part of the body around the lower ribs on the right side – should be stimulated by the application of alternate hot and cold packs and these may be used repeatedly because they are safe applications. Apply the hot pack over the liver area for two minutes. Immediately afterwards apply the cold pack for half a minute and continue in this way for ten minutes, finishing with the cold application.

The after-care of catarrhal jaundice is comparatively simple. By this time, however, the reader will be aware that in mucous colitis and jaundice of the most common type, there is within the system some mucoid material – usually surplus food material – which has formed catarrh, and so in passing it should be emphasized that the writer's book, *The Successful Treatment of Catarrh by Nature Cure Methods* (a companion book in this series), would repay careful study.

All starchy food should be taken in moderation, and milk and all protein foods, namely, meat, fish, fowl, eggs, cheese, peas, beans and lentils, should be curtailed as much as possible. The person with jaundice is one who *must* exercise; all movements are good, but brisk walking is the most effective. The cold waist compress, described in detail later in this book, can be applied with great benefit.

6.
Gall-Stones

THE TERM 'GALL-STONES' means that stonelike substances have formed in the gall-bladder or in its duct. This condition is much more common than is usually suspected and often, although these stones are present in quantity, no symptoms are recorded and they are frequently found after the death of the patient. It is also very interesting to note that the whole of the gall-bladder may be completely blocked by stone formation or by the presence of innumerable small stones without any sign of biliary colic, which is the most common symptom in this trouble. It seems incredible that this complete blockage of the gall-bladder can take place without any symptoms, and it must be assumed in such cases that the nervous system has become less sensitive.

Gall-stones are very rare under the age of thirty. They are usually found in females, especially those who have a sedentary occupation and who are inclined to be too stout and who have very lax abdominal walls. They are also more commen in women who suffer from chronic constipation. Pregnancy seems to be a factor and most of the women who suffer from this ailment have borne children. The trouble is also found very frequently where the diet has been one which has contained excessive starch and sugar and it is very interesting to note that gall-stones are less common where meat has been one of the staple articles of diet.

The presence of these stones is often discovered during X-ray examination of the liver and gall-bladder area, but when an attack of biliary colic occurs, then it is usual to suspect that gall-stones may be the cause.

BILIARY COLIC

Biliary colic is due to one or more gall-stones passing down the cystic duct and either going into the common bile duct or remaining lodged in the cystic duct or passing back into the gall-bladder. The pain is intense and agonizing and it occurs in paroxysms, usually in the region below the right ribs, but often radiating to the right shoulder. The patient is very much upset and there is vomiting, severe sweating and pallor, with jaundice often following, due to catarrhal inflammation caused by the irritation set up by the stone. The attack may last for a considerable time, but usually it is of short duration and there is an aching pain after the attack has subsided. Palpation often proves that the gall-bladder is distended. During the attack the temperature is high, often in the region of 102°, and the patient is generally very much upset. Jaundice is often absent when the cystic duct is the seat of the trouble.

It is difficult to offer a good reason for the onset of a biliary colic. Exercise or a sudden strain or indigestion may start the stone moving, and such an attack may be associated with a cleansing fast. The bowel motions should be studied after the attack, because often a quite big stone means inflammation at the bowel outlet. When the stone becomes impacted in the cystic duct, the gall-bladder swells and is readily palpated, but if the stone becomes impacted in the common bile duct, both the liver and gall-bladder can become enlarged, swollen and painful. Permanent jaundice may be the result. A number of attacks of biliary colic, even although they are of a mild nature, usually mean the presence of gall-stones.

One of the common results of the attempt of a gall-stone to pass down the ducts is suppuration. This may occur in the gall-bladder or in the common bile duct. The condition is serious in the gall-bladder because the stone may cause a rupture of the wall and this can lead to peritonitis. Suppuration in the bile ducts may cause rigor and general poisoning. An impacted gall-stone is very difficult to remove and frequently needs operation, although again Nature Cure methods, based on fasting, often bring about some movement of the stone.

THE TREATMENT OF GALL-STONES

During the actual attack of biliary colic, the patient should be fasted and given liberal amounts of warm water. The area around the lower ribs and upper abdomen on the right side should be treated by the application of alternate hot and cold packs. The hot pack, which consists of a folded cloth of several thicknesses, wrung out in very hot water, should be applied over the entire area for from one-and-a-half to two minutes. This should be followed by the application of a cloth or pack which has been soaked in cold water and wrung out. Continue in this alternate fashion until the sufferer gains relief. This simple method will give very good results in most cases but, as has been stated before, it is ineffective when the stone which has been attempting to move becomes impacted in one or other of the ducts or in the substance of the gall-bladder itself. After the attack has subsided, the patient usually feels sore and tight over the entire area of the gall-bladder and liver and this means that the application of the alternate hot and cold packs should be continued at regular intervals until this soreness disappears. In the meantime, the patient should be fasted as long as possible to enable the whole of the digestive system to be rested.

The person who has been told that she has gall-stones can do much to reduce these stones and prevent further formation. In the first instance, walking has a very beneficial action in the prevention of gall-stones and when a person is of stoutish build and inclined to over-eat of the starchy and fatty foods, then steps should be taken to reduce the weight as quickly as possible. Nothing will do this as effectively as the complete fast, taking only water. This may be continued for several days and it can be accompanied, if so desired, by the application of hot and cold packs. An even better plan during the fast, is to apply the hot and cold packs alternately for fifteen minutes, several times during the day, and at night to wear a high-waist cold compress. This will be described in detail in the chapter on water treatments. The cold compress is basically a treatment to increase circulation and drainage, and when applied to the waist area it will do much to increase the circulation and retone the muscles of all the vital organs.

There is a tendency for people who have gall-stones to have attacks during the cleansing fast. If this does occur, the fast should be taken very carefully and usually it is better to have a day or two on fresh acid fruit instead of water alone. Although these attacks of biliary colic do occur during fasting, this does not mean that it is a bad sign; it may be an uncomfortable one, but, without doubt, it is an indication of the cleansing which is being attempted by the body during the fasting stage. The person who is prone to the formation of gall-stones should seek a chart which describes the normal weight for his or her height and general build and endeavour to maintain the appropriate weight.

The diet in gall-stones must be very simple:

Breakfast — Fresh acid fruit such as apples, pears and oranges, with fruit juice.

Lunch — Vegetarian savoury or meat or steamed or baked fish or egg dish or cheese dish, with two steamed vegetables.

Dessert: Fruit or dates or raisins or sultanas or a junket.

Evening Meal — Salad of green and root vegetables with grated cheese: Wholewheat bread or crisp-bread.

Supper — Fruit only.

7.
Thrombosis and the Liver

IT WAS STATED at the beginning of this book that one of the weaknesses of the liver was that it had two blood supplies and therefore was subject to one of the common troubles of the times – thrombosis. Many liver ailments are caused by upsets of this nature, although the diagnosis is always difficult.

Thrombosis means the choking of an artery, complete or partial, with ultimate harm to the organ which is receiving the blood supply. It also means unhealthy, thickened and sluggish blood which can clot suddenly when it comes to a part of an artery which is already too congested. It is a trouble which does not occur in the healthy person even although that person is overworked and in a state of high emotional tension. The latter conditions do not in themselves cause thrombosis; there must be a thickened and sluggish blood-stream as a basic factor.

So, in spite of the many medical men who speak about thrombosis as 'the disease of modern times,' implying that it is due to the strain of life, this is not correct. It is a disease of insufficiency of certain substances in the food and also of excess of other substances which tend to create the thickened blood-stream.

One of the latter substances is called cholesterol and it is found in large quantities in the blood of the person suffering from thrombosis. There is definite proof that this is one of the main causes of the trouble, that is, an exciting cause which triggers off the reaction of the clotting. This substance is found in large quantities in certain foodstuffs and the following chart will give a rough idea of the amounts.

The amount of cholesterol in milligrams for each 100 grams:

Egg yolk	2,000
Lamb	610
Kidney	400
Butter	280
Cheese	160
Fish	190

It will be seen than an egg contains a large amount of cholesterol and the person · who has a thickened blood-stream with a tendency to upset of the liver function shown by the signs of poor general circulation would do well to eliminate eggs completely from the diet. This is the very first principle to follow before tackling the liver problem, because there are many cases of liver thrombosis of a partial nature.

DANGER OF TEA AND COFFEE

A dietetic point which is not fully understood is the danger of tea and coffee in the formation of the thrombotic bloodstream. People who take these beverages in large quantities nearly always have a high differential blood-pressure. The highest blood-pressure is recorded immediately next to the heart, or more exactly when the left ventricle of the heart has just contracted. This is called the systolic pressure and if it is too high there is danger of rupture of the wall of an artery. When the heart relaxes the lowest level of the human blood-pressure is recorded and this is called the diastolic pressure. The most important, however, is the difference between these two pressures, namely, the differential pressure. It is important because it shows the state of the arterial wall, and when the difference is greater than forty points it means that some of the elasticity has been lost. This is a most dangerous symptom, and if the bloodstream becomes thickened then the person is in danger of a thrombotic attack. Whenever possible a reading of the differential blood-pressure should be obtained from a practitioner.

It has been proved time and time again in records of patients and their diets that the heavy tea and coffee drinker tends nearly always to have some form of arterial hardening, shown by a high differential pressure. Therefore, if there is a tendency to poor circulation or if the differential is high, then the consumption of tea and coffee must be reduced to a very limited amount. These beverages are called 'social poisons' and their effect is similar. When first entering the blood-stream the liquid has the effect of thinning the blood and the person feels refreshed. This state may last for one or two hours, but gradually the blood again thickens and runs sluggishly. One other change has taken place. A certain amount of the drug contained in the tea or coffee has been transmitted to the wall of the artery. Gradually, repeated interchanges of this nature thicken the wall of the vessel and bring about the first arterial changes which cause the dreaded loss of elasticity. This is a very brief description of the harmful effects of these so-called mild poisons, and the reader will understand how the conditions are brought about which result in the arteries becoming so narrowed that thrombosis easily becomes a reality.

So far, in discussing the prevention of thrombosis, we have talked about the reduction of eggs and other foods which bring about the introduction of large amounts of cholesterol, and the danger of tea and coffee when taken in excess. If the sufferer stops taking these foods and liquids then the blood will commence to flow more vigorously. From this point we can build a diet which will do much to prevent blood-clotting.

DIET TO PREVENT THROMBOSIS

The first essential is always an adequate supply of vitamins in the daily diet. These are necessary to blood health, and the best breakfast for the person with thickened blood is a fruit one. Choose from sweet apples, pears, grapes, pineapple, grapefruit, and also the dried fruits. If liquid is required, then take some apple or orange juice or a glass of water. If a heavier breakfast is desired add some wholewheat cereal, and some wheat-germ. Lunch should be a mainly protein meal, but remember that eggs contain a large amount of cholesterol and take these very sparingly, say two per week. With the protein take two steamed vegetables and two jacketed potatoes. A fruit dessert is suitable if another course is desired, especially as there is reason to believe that fresh acid fruit provides a better digestive medium for the assimilation of protein foods. In people who are extremely thin, a wineglass of pineapple juice may be excellent as a dessert, because it activates the stomach juices.

The evening meal is difficult because most people think that another protein is required. If the differential blood-pressure is high, then this desire should be resisted, and a salad meal with wholewheat starch is indicated. If, however, there is no serious rise in the differential pressure, then a little protein in the form of cheese or grated nuts may be taken with salad and wholewheat starch.

This is an excellent diet for the person with a sluggish blood-stream, but there are also foods and liquids which must be curtailed. All demineralized foods leech minerals from the system and these include white sugar, white flour products, fried and greasy foods, condiments and preserves. These should be completely stopped and replaced when possible by wholesome compost-grown foods.

Once a diet is started, based upon the patient's understanding of its purpose, a remarkable change in the blood-stream will surely take place. This does not mean that the person will feel well immediately. Usually there is a considerable variation in the health. It may be excellent one day and the person may feel very sluggish the next. These are signs that the blood-stream is thinning and the impurities are being removed from the walls of the vessels and from storage areas. Real health is never stable, but when the blood-stream is clean then a person may experience a standard of health which can never be appreciated at any other time. As the blood-stream thins then the person really becomes alive and the danger of thrombotic blockage of the liver blood-vessels is completely removed. This is a very definite statement, but to every action there is an equal and positive reaction and arterial health can be expected when the right foods and liquids are taken.

DANGER OF NEGATIVE EMOTIONS

It is not correct, however, to think that that is all there is to thrombosis. Other important points must be studied. This trouble affects mainly the business man, who is continually beset by tension, worry and emotional upsets and these can definitely affect blood-pressure, raising it rapidly far above the normal. The more frequently the pressure is raised in this way, the more tendency there is for it to become too high and remain at this level. In other words, it does not quickly return to normal. Worry often leads to the negative emotion of violent anger. This also causes poisons to form in the blood-stream which, because of their very nature, cannot be dealt with by the liver. The walls of the arteries become scarred and thickened and lose their elasticity. Negative emotions of this kind must be avoided. The diet outlined helps to calm the person, but understanding of the danger of anger will also help.

WALKING FOR ACTIVE CIRCULATION

The person who lives in his business, and often calls it his hobby, seldom gets sufficient exercise to keep the circulation active. This is really vital; motor cars are so handy that exercise is usually confined to an occasional round of golf. Such a person would be much less liable to the thrombotic attack if he walked a certain distance each day. Walking is the best of all forms of exercise because it stimulates the leg circulation. It is not generally known that the drainage of the legs is not so much due to heart action as to the movement of the muscles of the legs, and an efficient circulation in the legs and feet does much to remove the tendency to clotting in the liver circulation.

Eat carefully, control the emotions, and walk every day; these are the three golden rules for the person who has been warned by symptoms pointing to thrombosis.

8.
General Diet for Liver Health

IT IS OUR birthright to be healthy and, although we are not all born so, if we progress correctly we should have clean tissues and a fair degree of health when we reach adult age. This is a profound Nature Cure belief and many practitioners have written about the methods whereby this can be accomplished. People who read these writings soon appreciate that the healthy child can easily become the healthy adult. The child, however, who is born sickly, can usually, by good diet and general hygiene, also achieve comparatively healthy adulthood and, indeed, many live to a very ripe old age. Once a healthy state has been achieved, it is our duty to retain it by studying nature's laws and obeying the sound principles of living.

The person suffering from liver and its associated troubles has made mistakes in his or her life. Most of these mistakes are due to lack of knowledge and it is our duty at this time to outline how they can be corrected. The body always tends to heal because there is within it a force of positiveness, a buoyancy which brings correction of imperfection. Once this is appreciated then the reader will understand that we must attempt to find out what the body is trying to do and assist it in every way possible.

EMOTIONS AFFECT BODY RHYTHM

Generally speaking, if a person is in good mental health, is happy and contented, then his body's mechanism works comparatively easily and the amount of impurity is not allowed to accumulate. If, however, a person becomes mentally ill or emotionally distressed in any way, then there is a tendency for the body to lose its rhythm, to become unbalanced and to work less efficiently. So, first of all, it must be stressed that everyone seeking the cure for liver troubles or any trouble mentioned in this book should attempt to understand what happens in the body and also to appreciate that every effort must be made to relieve any emotional ill-health.

No system of cure can be complete unless it recognizes the influence upon the body exerted by the human mind. Modern conditions strain the individual very much but usually more on the emotional level than the physical. Anger, jealousy, fear, and many other conditions are very often mirrored in the various physical signs such as palpitation, shortness of breath and loss of weight, and it is very difficult to draw a dividing line between emotional distress and actual physical conditions. So every reader of this book should search his mind for any disturbance which is upsetting the normal rhythm of the body. Most people know that they have become upset emotionally, but usually it is difficult to decide exactly when the upset took place. Frequently it has been present long before the incident which is usually blamed for the upset. In other words, people become emotionally unstable over a period of time without actually realizing it. Then a certain happening takes place in which they are really upset and this is blamed as the causative factor, but actually they have not been too well for a considerable period beforehand.

Now this is not a thing that can be treated alone and it is much better if a Nature Cure practitioner, who is skilled in these occurrences, or a psychologist or even a very sincere friend is brought in to discuss this matter, to bring it right up to date and to show it in a new light. From this angle it is usually possible to correct the emotional upset which is causing the stagnation of the vital organs around the centre of the body. This is the most difficult part of the treatment, and patience and care are usually necessary before a person who is not on a normal thinking level can be led back gradually to where he actually left the path, but it is wonderful what a free discussion can accomplish in this connection.

Now, outside of emotional conditions, it is often found that the basic physical complaint has been brought about by a very poor system of dieting. Many people argue that diet is unimportant and generally the ordinary medical practitioner does not pay too much attention to this aspect. With more experience, however, it becomes obvious that people are divided into types, that each type has a definite digestive weakness, and that certain foods, if taken in excess, or of poor quality, will cause ill-health in that person. This does not mean that ill-health will always occur in the digestive system. First, therefore, we have to find out generally which type of food should be taken and which should be avoided by the person who suffers from liver and associated ailments.

PROTEINS STRAIN LIVER

The liver, as has been stated before, is a very complicated organ, and, like all such organs, it can go wrong rather easily. So it would appear to be a very good plan to arrange the diet so that the liver is not given too much work to do, and so that food is not taken in very peculiar mixtures. The foods which cause the greatest strain on the liver are the protein foods, such as meat, fish, fowl, eggs and cheese. Other foods, of course, are dealt with by the liver too, but the proteins are the ones which throw the greatest strain on the digestive part of this very complex organ which has a lot of work to do in other directions. So we should attempt to build a diet with fewer proteins.

Various statements have been made that the liver requires meat proteins to get full working capacity and that certain people are anaemic because these are not given. Most of us know, however, of vegetarians who dispense absolutely with all forms of flesh foods and who live healthily and have a very efficiently acting liver. There are difficulties in the vegetarian diet, make no mistake about that, but it would appear that moderation in all things is what is required and in the diet about to be described, we have aimed at moderation. Liver trouble or the tendency to it is already present and here we are not faced with any herculean task, but just a sensible way of building up the action of the liver.

LOW-PROTEIN DIET

The diet must, of necessity, be light and there is no better way to ensure this than by making the first meal of the day as meagre as possible. Now most people think that to start off with a very light breakfast is not very pleasant, but Nature Cure is a system based on personal effort. Nothing is *given* to the body; it depends on the desire of the patient to get well and his ability to carry out the axioms as carefully as possible. Some people may say, 'Oh, I couldn't take a breakfast which has no protein.' This, of course, is ridiculous. Many, many thousands of people in this world do very heavy manual work without taking a protein for breakfast.

Breakfast — If the abdominal trouble is severe, then breakfast may be missed completely and only a glass of warm water need be taken, especially if the tongue is coated. Certain people find that fruit juices are more suitable and grape, lemon or apple juice can be taken, although in other cases it is found that fruit juice appears to be too much acid in its effect. When the condition is not acute, fruit of any kind such as an apple or pear or dried fruit, can be taken with the addition of wheat-germ. Others find that they cannot live on fruit alone and these people should take a breakfast of fruit, either fresh or dried, with some cereal.

Such a breakfast is quite satisfying and yet it does not overload. It gives sufficient energy without throwing a great deal of work on the liver and so digestion is easily accomplished and the body is not clogged in any way. Now this is most important, because over-loading of the body is one of the most common findings in liver and like troubles and here we have a very good breakfast which can be easily digested, assimilated and finally eliminated without any great strain on the system. Such a breakfast would be wasted by introducing an egg, or some form of cheese or some other protein, and it is advisable therefore to keep to the fruit, fruit juices and cereal. There are certain writers who believe that the acid fruits and starches do not really mix, believing that the initial digestion of starch in the mouth, where it should turn to a form of sugar, is prevented by the taking of acid fruit and there are many people who find that such a mixture is not ideal. In these cases, the acid fruits, oranges, grapefruit, etc., should be stopped and dried fruit and cereal taken instead. Other people find that they are not suitable subjects for dried fruit and prefer to take rough wholewheat bread or wholewheat toast instead and this is also allowable, but the more starch that is taken the more the strain on the liver.

Second Meal — The person suffering from liver troubles should have one golden rule — that one meal daily should consist of a large raw salad composed of green and root vegetables which have been grated and prepared just before being served. With this, take nothing but starchy food, e.g., crispbread, with butter and perhaps a little honey. Olive oil and lemon juice in small amounts are preferable to the proprietary types of salad dressing.

Third Meal — The third meal, the meal in which the protein dish is taken, may present some difficulty. Start with vegetable soup. This should not be made with meat stock, but with one of the well-known vegetarian flavouring agents. If meat is taken, then it should not be provided more frequently than twice weekly. Fish should be introduced once weekly at the most. Eggs, lightly cooked, should be taken three times per week, and on the other days a vegetarian savoury dish should compose the basic part of the meal. Now with this protein it is necessary to take two or three green and root vegetables and potatoes baked in their jackets, especially if the savoury itself is not too starchy. Some of the vegetarian dishes tend to be starchy and there is no need then for the baked potatoes. For sweet, if desired, have fresh or dried fruit, such as raisins or sultanas, or a milk jelly. For supper, the last meal of the day, it is always advisable to keep to fruit only and usually fresh acid fruit is best.

It is unlikely that a diet based on the above will suit everyone and in some cases stomach acidity will occur. This may be due to one particular food or to certain food mixtures and only the person involved can find this out. Careful note-taking will soon reveal the offending food, which should then be kept out of the diet.

9.
Water Treatments

IN NATURE CURE establishments water treatments are used largely to stimulate skin action and to improve the circulation of the blood and lymphatic streams. Naturally this demands apparatus and it puts many of the treatments outside the scope of the person who is conducting the treatment at home. There are, however, many simple methods of using water which can help the person suffering from liver and kindred disorders.

Peculiarly enough, the first and most important water treatment is not directed at the abdominal area but at the entire skin. To understand this it should be explained that the person suffering from liver complaints is really suffering from an excess of unnatural substances in his blood-stream, and these must be removed via the eliminating organs, i.e., the lungs, kidneys, bowels and skin. The latter tissue then becomes very important and must be stimulated into activity. This does not mean that the skin is necessarily inactive, but steps must be taken to ensure that it is doing its part.

To ensure skin activity the entire body should be rubbed with a rough towel until it becomes pink and glowing. This is an effective treatment because many of the dead cells are removed and the skin becomes thin and moveable and is more active in expressing impurities. It is a treatment which can be carried out by anyone even when in a very weak state. The application of hot water to the skin is not advised because it tends to weaken skin action, and the tissue may lose tone if too many hot baths are taken.

COLD SKIN RUBS

In the vital person cold baths have a totally different reaction and they are recommended to all who suffer from liver trouble, provided the reaction is good. When cold water is applied to the skin the sensation of chill is recorded in the brain and immediately more blood is sent to the part. This results in a washing away of impurities and a feeding of the tissues by the increased flow of fresh blood. Cold water bathing also means that the skin receives a friction rub and this further creates the ideal covering of a thin, dry skin which reacts to all changes in temperature, expresses impurities in large amounts and relieves the strain placed on the other organs of elimination.

So the best water treatment to begin with is the cold sponge down. Do this in a warm bathroom. Apply the water all over the body with the hands and finish by rubbing the entire skin dry with the hands. This is much better than drying with a towel. The cold bath is an even better treatment, but naturally it requires that the person be young and vigorous to enable the body to again warm up quickly. These baths, however, have a very beneficial effect when these requirements are present and can help to relieve quickly any form of liver congestion. A good reaction means that the body becomes red and glowing after the cold bath and the person feels good and does not have a chilly feeling some time later. Many people shun cold water treatment in any form, however, and it is useless to advise them to take such treatment. It is also unwise to continue with cold water treatment if there is not a good reaction, because a severe chill may result.

LOCAL WATER TREATMENTS

The foregoing treatments are of a general nature, their

purpose being to increase the whole of the circulation and to improve the drainage of the body. The best local treatments for liver trouble are the sitz bath and the cold compress.

The sitz or hip bath is one in which the patient sits in water, splashing it upwards over the abdomen and having the feet and the rest of the body clear of the water. There are special baths designed for this purpose, but the ordinary one can be used if the person sits in the bath in such a way that the feet are supported at the end.

In the cold sitz bath some ten inches of cold water is required. The hips are immersed and the water splashed over the abdomen. This bath should be of very short duration and should last only some thirty seconds, and the hips and thighs must then be dried thoroughly. It is an excellent way of regaining the circulation of the abdomen and does much to strengthen the liver, but the patient *must* feel invigorated after such a bath, otherwise it is too severe for him. For instance, if such a bath is taken and the patient feels well, but within a few hours the feet become cold and the person feels listless, then a cold sitz bath is too strenuous for the vitality of that patient or else the duration of the bath has been too long. This is a most important point. If the patient feels well and has no unpleasant after-effects, then the cold sitz bath can be used frequently by the person who is following a Nature Cure régime in an effort to control and cure liver troubles.

The water treatment which suits most people is compressing. This is an age-old method of applying water with the express purpose of stimulating the arterial, venous and lymphatic systems. Compressing is always effective when the desired reaction is obtained, but there are several contra-indications which must be studied.

Firstly, this method is not successful if the patient feels that water treatment in any form makes his condition worse. This point is not always stressed in Nature Cure literature, but there are people who always have ill-effects after any form of water treatment and in such cases compressing is not advised.

Compressing is not suitable just before or during the menstrual period, and it is not advised when the patient is very weak or extremely tired. This method needs quite a vital reaction and therefore the patient must have a fair degree of residual strength. On the other hand, compressing is best in its effect on fevers or when the nervous system of the body is very irritated. Its soothing powers can be remarkable and it is one of the greatest aids to the person who suffers from sleeplessness.

TECHNIQUE

The cold compress used in liver and allied ailments is arranged as follows: a piece of linen is cut about eight to ten inches broad and of a length to go once round the waist and overlap about two inches for fastening. It should be one layer thick unless ordered otherwise by the practitioner. The linen is soaked thoroughly in cold water, wrung out and applied round the waist and fastened with safety pins. It should be wound fairly tightly on the body and then covered with several layers of warm, dry material, such as flannel. The flannel should completely cover the linen, overlapping it in every way.

Normally, compresses are applied before the sufferer retires for the night. If the reaction is satisfactory, they are kept on the body all night and usually they are completely dry in the morning. The reaction desired is that the linen, which at first is cold and clammy, becomes comfortably warm. This can be ascertained by slipping the fingers between the skin and the linen. This reaction should occur within half-an-hour of the compress being applied. Usually by this time the patient will have fallen asleep and this means that the reaction is good.

If, however, the linen does not heat up, the compress should be removed and the skin rubbed down with a rough towel to increase the circulation and remove any local chilling. It is impossible to tell when a compress is going to work properly and a person can compress successfully for months and then suddenly, without any warning, a reaction fails to occur.

Compresses should normally be worn five nights weekly. The linen should be removed and boiled after every application and the skin of the area covered by the compress should be washed with warm, soapy water.

10.

Exercises

IT HAS BEEN said that liver troubles mainly effect those people who are fair, fat and forty and there is certainly some truth in this statement. These troubles are founded on congestion, and physical activity is required to reduce congestion. The person who suffers in this way is usually over-weight, seldom goes for energetic walks and, if exercise is taken at all, it is usually very spasmodic because tiredness afterwards is extreme. Gradually, active movements are avoided. Others, at the start of the trouble, note that they feel better after exercise and they persist until the condition becomes so bad that they are forced to give up. If what has been written in this book has been studied carefully and the advice has been followed, then the time has come for the sufferer from liver trouble to study the value of again exercising the body.

The best of all exercise is walking. Walk as briskly as possible, keeping the legs straight and having the clothing light and free-fitting. This may result in rapid tiring of the physical body and the person is often forced to slow down. The walk should be concluded before real fatigue sets in. Next day the same performance should be gone through and again the walk should be ended before the person becomes too tired. Walking should be gradually lengthened as strength is gained. After each walk sponge the body down with warm, soapy water, and if there is a good reaction, finish with a cold sponge down and a brisk friction rub. Such exercise will result in a general improvement of the whole body and the liver action will be greatly invigorated. Many people cannot get enough interest in walking, thinking it a waste of time, and so golf, tennis, bowls, gardening and fishing or any such recreation becomes invaluable to get the organs around the abdominal area really working. Exercise is life to the person suffering from this ailment.

At the same time it will usually be found that the tiredness which comes after unaccustomed exercise is really overwhelming and that is why the baths and friction rubs are so helpful. If desired, a full hot bath may be taken occasionally to ease the strained muscles, but, generally speaking, such a bath is too relaxing.

Next to walking, side-bending exercises are the best stimulant to the liver circulation. Here is one which is very useful. Stand erect with the hands on the waist, thumbs to the back pressing behind the lower ribs. Now bend sharply to the right, pressing in with the right hand towards the spine. Straighten the body and again bend as far as possible to the right. Now straighten the body and bend sharply to the left, pressing inwards towards the spine with the left hand. This is the complete sequence of the exercise. Bend twice to the right in succession and once to the left. This brings about a definite squeezing of the organs in the area and greatly aids the blood-flow.

The same exercise can be made more strenuous by the following variations. Stand erect with the feet apart. Raise the arms straight above the head. Now turn the body slightly to the left and attempt to touch the left foot with the hands. This throws a great strain on the right side. Now straighten the body, with the hands still above the head, and bend to the right side, attempting to touch the right foot with the hands. Continue in this alternate fashion until slightly tired.

LIVER BEATING

It has been found, during the study of organic re-actions, that beating over the liver area with the clenched fist causes a reduction in the size of the organ and forces the bile into the bile duct. This is best done in the following position: stand leaning slightly forward with the feet wide apart. Now, using the clenched fist, beat fairly solidly and rhythmically on the right ribs at the back, below the shoulder blade. The beating must not be too heavy otherwise it may harm the ribs, but it must be firm. About twenty beats are enough and will result in a considerable feeling of uplift if the liver has been badly congested. Some people will find it difficult to get enough power into the blow to make much difference and they should enlist the services of a friend or go to a Nature Cure practitioner to have the action correctly performed. Guidance on this exercise is most helpful.

DIAPHRAGM EXERCISE

Lie on the back with the knees up and place a book on the abdomen just below the lower ribs. Now breathe in, in such a way that the book is raised a considerable distance. Notice that this must be achieved through breathing and not by muscular action. At first it will be impossible in many cases to make the diaphragm move sufficiently downwards to raise the abdominal structures, but with practice this will be achieved and again the benefit of the internal massage of the liver area is of value. This diaphragmatic exercise should be practised at first for some five minutes daily, but gradually the time should be increased until at least fifteen minutes either at once or at different periods during the day is spent exercising in this way.

Usually it is better to perform these exercises on rising and before retiring. It is common to find that the body and its muscles are stiff in the morning, but a few movements should bring back mobility.

It should be noted that the side-bending exercises get considerable movement in the spine between the shoulder blades and the hips. This is a most important part because the nerves which leave the spine in this area affect the abdominal organs and very often the spine is very tight in this area. It cannot be expected that full movement will be immediately regained, but with practice it will improve until a very full range is obtained. Keep practising these spinal movements until it is felt that the liver can be squeezed in the side-bending. This is a form of self-massage and can be most useful in promoting liver health. Remember that liver troubles are not common in the very active, mainly due to the continual invigoration. So, become active, even if it is against all inclination.

Talking about spinal movement brings to mind the great value of osteopathy in this connection. Most registered naturopaths practise this method and manipulation of the neck and thoracic bones can have a very beneficial effect on liver conditions. In most cases these spinal joints are stiffened without the patient being aware of this trouble. Manipulation of this nature is never severe when the muscles and ligaments of the spinal area are bound and contracted. Forcible movement would tear, and so the practitioner spends considerable time with heat treatments, deep tissue massage and exercise before he locks one part of the spine and moves the other part to get the joint movement he requires.

Results after this can be quite spectacular, especially if the person is living on as natural and as balanced a diet as can be obtained. Dieting alone will release tightened muscles which are continually being fed from an impure, acid blood-stream. Generally speaking, however, quicker results can be obtained by manipulation and massage.

Other books for better health the natural way.

SLEEPLESSNESS

Its Prevention and Cure by Natural Methods

Cyril Scott

Most people resort to drugs when they are afflicted by sleeplessness but the majority of cases require no medicinal remedies, being caused by faulty habits of living which can be corrected by following the natural therapies provided in this book. Author includes biochemic and homoeopathic prescriptions, with notes on their individual characteristics. Every method described is utterly safe and non-toxic.

HERBAL CURES OF DUODENAL ULCER AND GALL STONES

Frank Roberts

Neither surgery nor chemicals can *cure* an ulcer; at best they only temporarily alleviate painful symptoms. But the herbal remedies given in this book offer a permanent cure. Author's simple treatments have brought relief to many thousands of sufferers. He includes details of a sure method for the elimination of gall stones within twenty-four hours.

CANCER PREVENTION

Fallacies and Some Reassuring Facts

Cyril Scott

The 'fallacies' include the belief that radium and surgery can 'cure' cancer, while the 'reassuring facts' feature homoeopathic achievements, the grape cure, and a simple preventive measure which will encourage every reader. This sane and intelligent book removes much of the dread born of many misunderstandings surrounding the subject of cancer.